Impressum / legal notice

© Copyright 2019

1. Auflage / 1. Edition
Kontakt / contact:

Fernando Carrillo Castillo

Am Fackelstein 3a

56305 Puderbach, Germany

Covergestaltung / cover design:

Fernando Carrillo Castillo

Made in the USA
Las Vegas, NV
03 December 2020